Learning to Cope

Helen Good Brenneman

HERALD PRESS
Scottdale, Pennsylvania
Kitchener, Ontario

LEARNING TO COPE

Copyright © 1975 by Herald Press, Scottdale, Pa. 15683
  Published simultaneously in Canada by Herald Press,
  Kitchener, Ont. N2G 1A7
Library of Congress Catalog Card Number: 75-32724
International Standard Book Number: 0-8361-1782-4
Printed in the United States of America
Design by Alice B. Shetler

To those who would soar high above the treetops, but find that because of a broken wing they must settle for green pastures and the warmth of the sun upon the earth, this book is empathetically dedicated.

CONTENTS

Preface 9
1. Polish Your Self-Image 15
2. The School of Patience 21
3. She Digs the Earth 27
4. Mountains to Climb 40
5. Through Sunlight and Shadow 48
6. From Wheelchair to Pike's Peak ... 54
7. When God Does Not Heal 59
8. Professional Advice from a
   Paralyzed Psychiatrist 68
9. The Uses of Adversity 76
The Author 85

PREFACE

I remember the happy day the word "cope" became an important part of my outlook on life. Since then I have tried to keep this word before my eyes when the inconveniences of being partially handicapped made life's journey bumpy and uneven, both literally and figuratively. Concentrating on this good four-letter word has helped me think of possible solutions to my many dilemmas.

The word first burst into my consciousness when I called a friend on the telephone and asked her how she was making it. Geri walked with crutches because of an earlier bout with polio, but held a responsible part-time job. (See Chapter Four.) Geri's brief and ready reply was, "Well, I'm coping."

This, of course, did not mean that Geri had no problems or that she was always able to cope. She could tell you, just as I can, of many occasions when we have not successfully coped despite our good intentions. But the thought, "I'm coping," makes us feel we are on top of a situation rather than the victim of circumstances.

On the other hand, I read the account of someone with a handicap who "coped" by bluffing his way along, never really facing the situation with which he had to deal. This is a misuse of the word.

One Sunday when my husband was out of the country on a business trip, I met a friend after church and we engaged in a lighthearted conversation. I told her that when the other members of the family were all away I often made myself TV dinners. However, I explained, there was one drawback. Because of my poor vision, I once put a dinner into a 250-degree oven and half an hour later discovered it was still cold. So now I always turn the oven up, by guess, whether it needs it or not.

"Well, why on earth don't you call me at times like that?" she asked.

"Oh, I save such calls for real emergencies," I replied. "Besides, I try to live by the word 'cope.'"

"There's another word to consider," she countered. "It's the word 'pride.'"

Now that was food for thought. I know we must swallow our pride at times. For example, this book was written in spite of a severe visual problem. I would not have been able to complete it without my friends who volunteered their services to be "eyes" for me. But I still want to be able to cope when I can.

Another angle on the word "cope" is that we

can't do it in our own strength. A friend once remarked that the letters in the word might stand for "*Christ Our Peace Evermore.*" Perhaps God is trying to say something to us through our difficulties. Spiritually, we can "run and not be weary and walk and not faint." Our spiritual perception is not limited by the state of our optical nerves, nor cataracts, nor nearsightedness. We can *hope* that God will be glorified in situations where we cannot *cope*.

This book is written both for my own edification (it speaks to my personal need) and to share inspiration with others who are going through similar experiences. Our problems are as varied as our personal appearance, and the same disease may manifest itself in a multitude of ways.

After I wrote an article about my young friend, Jane, which I have included as Chapter 6 in this book ("From Wheelchair to Pike's Peak"), my children wondered why I too could not learn to take somersaults and dispense with my wheelchair. I almost wished I had not written the article! To compare our symptoms, handicaps, and ability to cope, is not too helpful. But we can inspire one another to live life to its fullest within our particular limitations.

Although this book is written in the context of the physically handicapped, of whom there are many, I hope it will also speak to those with less visible handicaps and limitations. For all of us have some handicap, and sometimes the invisible ones cause the greater hurt. There are emotional limitations, often through no fault of our own — inferiority complexes, feelings of inadequacy, emotional limps. There are spiritual problems — guilt that has not been resolved, loss of brotherhood in crucial life experiences, misunderstanding and misappropriation of the grace of a loving God.

I hope, also, that this book will promote understanding of the special problems of persons with handicaps which box us in when we face the challenges and adventures of life.

I hesitate to give much specific advice. My doctor friend tells me that a major problem of the handicapped and the parents of handicapped children is the abundance of advice from well-meaning friends. Such unsolicited counsel often creates more problems than it solves.

I profited about as much from the words of my three-year-old neighbor, Jeff, as from the suggestions of many adult friends. After he had asked many questions, I explained that "the muscles in my legs just don't work very well." Looking at me with all the experience and wisdom of his years, he advised, "I eat Wheaties."

At least he didn't come back to check on whether I had taken his advice.

Anything I have written in this book must be applied to the peculiar circumstances of the person who reads it. And I promise not to check on how well you are "coping."

I am deeply grateful to the publishers who granted permission to reprint from their periodicals some of the chapters in this book and to Bertha Bender and Elizabeth Bender who graciously read the manuscript.

— *Helen Good Brenneman*

POLISH YOUR
SELF-IMAGE

ON THE children's television program, *Sesame Street*, Big Bird said he was feeling pretty ordinary; but when he happened to look into the mirror he saw a Very Special Bird.

Those of us who live with a handicap — and who doesn't have one kind or another — would benefit from doing the same. If we look into the mirror, we will see a Very Special Bird, special with God because of His love and acceptance of us and of our own particular place in His scheme of things.

Our self-image and sense of "personhood" often take a real beating when we are limited by physical and emotional handicaps. Although the Apostle Paul wrote that we should not think too highly of ourselves, it is also clear that we should not depreciate ourselves. For the rest of that verse in Romans 12 goes on to say that we should think with sober judgment. And Phillips helps us by wording the Scripture this way: "Don't cherish exaggerated ideas of yourself or your importance, but try to have a sane estimate of your capabilities by the light of the faith that God has given to you all."

It would not hurt any of us to polish up our self-images a bit. In fact, our families might find us easier to live with! For those of us with handicaps, this means that we accept ourselves with both our limitations and our special gifts. Someone has said, "Self-acceptance is the beginning of change."

The following suggestions are not conclusive, but are simply ideas I have had simmering on the back burner of my mind. Frankly, I am writing them down for myself. You may want to add some ideas of your own.

As Paul says, *evaluate your strengths and weaknesses*, arriving at a reasonable estimate of your capabilities. Recently, I attended a women's retreat where each participant was presented with a questionnaire based on the Sermon on the Mount to be filled out in some quiet place. Some of the questions brought me up short. "Do you think you have been given any gifts which, if not hidden, can lead others to glorify

God?" "What do you like about yourself — what do you dislike?"

Soon after this retreat I noticed that the Apostle Paul, writing an epistle to fellow Christians, began his letter, "Paul, called by the will of God to be an apostle of Christ Jesus. . . ." I wondered, if I were to begin a letter in that way, what would I write? "Helen, called by the will of God to be a helpmate, a mother, an encourager, a friend . . .?" How do I evaluate my call?

Paul also writes that we should "stir up the gift of God that is in us." We are not to despise God's gifts to us — we are to use them.

Develop hobbies and interests within your own particular limitations. We are usually capable of accomplishing much more than we do. Not long after I had a battle with serious illness, a wise pastor called on me. Instead of suffocating me with sympathy, he made a rather heavy assignment — to edit the monthly parish newssheet. For me this was a kind of "resurrection," for I discovered that I could carry out a job which was dear to my heart. Also, I found myself back in the ebb and flow of the work of the church.

I remember my mother telling a story from her own school days. A certain student, Susan, answered every challenge with the words, "I can't." One day the teacher wrote on the blackboard, "Susan can't." In contrast to that, Paul wrote, "I can do all things through Christ who strengthens me." All things, that is, which Christ wants me to do.

Accept limitations as matter-of-factly as possible. As a victim of multiple sclerosis, I have a variety of problems and handicaps which are quite conspicuous and difficult to ignore. Sometimes I feel like a combination of the lame, the halt, and the blind!

I have often wondered how much I should talk about these things to others. When are people genuinely interested in my condition, and when are they just being polite?

I think honest, interested questions deserve honest, matter-of-fact answers. When we are not afraid to say, "Please excuse me, I must take a nap," or "Just go ahead, it takes me a while to go down stairs," I believe we put other people more at ease.

Make a list of problems caused by your handicaps and limitations. This might include such things as getting ready for church on time (when a bathroom is shared by numerous members of a family) or avoiding spillage when carrying dishes from the table. Work out ways of coping — perhaps getting counsel from visiting nurses, rehabilitation specialists, or friends — and develop a fairly regular routine.

Some solutions are so simple we wonder why they did not occur to us before. My visual handicap is partially relieved by a magnifying glass with a light, obtained from a local optometrist. But it was located on the desk in my bedroom. Every time I wished to read a recipe or the directions on a cleaning bottle, I made a trip into the bedroom. It occurred to me that a magnifying glass in the kitchen would put an end to this nonsense, and a ninety-five cent purchase solved the problem.

Carry out the necessary procedures with simplicity and quiet dignity. To keep our self-images in good shape, we should avoid apologizing (which makes everyone uncomfortable), complaining (even though we do feel a little sorry for ourselves), or acting as though we don't care (when, of course, we do).

A more subtle temptation is to overcompensate by exaggerating other accomplishments. I remember a homemaker who always said, "I can't sew, but I can cook." To cover up her sense of inadequacy in one field, she needed to point out her proficiency in another.

Stay in the mainstream of life as much as possible. A child I knew developed a seemingly incurable disease but she was not satisfied to sit on the sidelines of life and indulge in "invalidism." Jane fought her disease with daily exercises and insisted on joining her schoolmates in as many activities as her physical condition would allow.

We may not be able to take part in all the activities we would enjoy, but we can at least remain curious and interested. Foolish pride often causes us to withdraw from life.

Remain curious and interested in life, enjoying the people who come your way. I have noticed that when one loses a faculty such as vision, one learns to sharpen another, such as the ability to listen. The world is filled with people who long for a listening ear. One of the best ways to keep from becoming self-centered is to take an active interest in others, listening, praying, and sharing.

A few years ago I read a letter to the editor of a large Boston paper. The writer responded to a question from another reader, "Can anyone help an MS victim?" and she signed her letter "Knotty Knees." She gave some very good advice:

"If anyone asks how you feel, don't tell them, but answer, "Good, great, haven't felt so well in years,'then change the subject immediately and ask how they are. You may have to listen to many ailments, but they have long since forgotten their question to you. . . . Only you know how you feel, and sad as it may seem, when it boils right down to it, only you can do anything about it. I often offer my slightest pain or deepest hurt up to God. . . . I always tell the guests coming that it's a strictly self-service affair and someone will even have to wait on me, but they can pull straws or toss a penny on that one. Your true friends won't care, even if the cup and saucer don't match, or if your coffee turns out rotten, or your tea is too strong. Your true friends are happy if you are, and isn't it amazing to find out who they are?"

Knotty Knees took a realistic look at herself when she glanced in the mirror, but she had a healthy self-image. For she also saw a Very Special Person, with special gifts, not the least of which was friendliness.

THE SCHOOL OF PATIENCE

I ALWAYS thought I would return to college after the children were grown, but I didn't expect to get my education this way. The other day I remarked to a friend, "I am working on my MS in Patience and I'm not sure I'll pass."

Unfortunately, I do not mean my Master of Science degree, for MS — to *me* — stands for "Multiple Sclerosis." And the laboratory where I worked on my problems was a household with my husband and four growing children. I began this curriculum more than ten years ago, and the tuition is high. As mother of four children ranging in years from six to twelve, I had been active in home, church, and community life in our small Midwestern town. One day I discovered that I could not run. Other strange frightening symptoms appeared, disappeared, and appeared again.

But it was not until we spent a year in Boston, where my husband was studying under a grant, that matters became really bad. Suddenly I found myself a patient in Massachusetts General Hospital, almost completely helpless. My legs were irresponsive. They refused to hold me up or to obey my brain when I ordered them to move. My right hand became spastic and my left hand partially so. It was frustrating not to be able to comb my hair, write to my parents, or even to feed myself in an acceptable way.

The doctors could not promise that I would respond to the drugs they were giving me, and those were difficult days. But they were also days of comfort, for friends around the world sent messages that they were praying to God for us. Their prayers were answered, for after a month of hospitalization I was at home once more with my family. I had learned to walk all over again. My hands were not yet functioning well, but they gradually improved and I was soon able to do a limited amount of work and use my electric typewriter.

For several years we had run our household by teamwork, for I had taken on a part-time job when my husband returned to graduate school. But the children had not needed to carry so much responsibility as they now had to assume. During my absence, my husband, a good organizer and a consistent disciplinarian, had regulated life in our apartment. Now I was there, unable to do much physical work but able to see when it didn't get done!

My patience, which has always been on the skimpy side, was taxed to the limit by my junior partners, who didn't see things as I did. My thirteen-year-old daughter liked to arrange her own schedule, and I didn't blame her. She didn't want me harping at her the minute she walked in the door.

At our country home in Indiana I used to write instructions on a blackboard, and I found that the children took my suggestions better that way than by the spoken word. But in our Boston apartment I had no blackboard. Even to my own ears, my words sounded like nagging.

I shared with my prayer group my besetting sin of impatience.

"Yes," one of my friends responded, "I know just what you mean. My sister became incapacitated and nearly drove the rest of us crazy, even though we were adults. When she wanted something picked up, she wanted it done right then. Finally, we just told her off."

This testimonial helped me to visualize myself as my family might see me — a demanding invalid lying on a couch. I prayed, "Lord, save me from invalidism!"

He enabled me to do a number of routine chores, in addition to several hours of desk work each day. I still relied heavily on younger members of the family to operate vacuums, rake leaves, and help in the kitchen. But I learned to make schedules of long-term responsibilities, write out lists of chores that change from day to day, and block out the children's working time so that I did not have to be continually interrupting them.

I'm not a bit apologetic that my children learned responsibility. I would be far more reluctant to send a daughter into the world who could not make a casserole or keep a house reasonably clean or take care of her laundry. Nor would I want to launch a son who could not work with his hands as well as his mind. I tell my children that even had I not become handicapped, I would not have raised them to be helpless. Work is a part of normal life.

I soon learned that I must choose outside activities with care. If a particular PTA meeting was of special importance, I had to take it easy that afternoon in order to attend. And this limitation of time and energy has made me wonder if all the meetings couples usually attend are really that important. How can we make our homelife more enjoyable if we are always on the run, tensely keyed to our clocks and calendars?

Sometimes our children benefited by what we weren't able to do for them. Since I was no longer able to drive and had no driver's license, I could not chauffeur the children to their many destinations. My husband did more than his share of this, but the children learned to go to the doctors' offices, stores, school affairs, and church events on their bicycles or on their own good feet. We feel our children gained self-reliance as they took care of their transportation and went out alone.

Being at home much of the time, I had to fight the temptation to "overmother" my children. I am sure I would have been a far more domineering wife and mother if I had had no consuming interest of my own. When the children were small, I took the advice of friends and developed my interest in writing in spite of the affairs of the busy years. Now this avocation is a window for my soul.

When a grievous circumstance comes to one member of the family, it affects all the others, though the one who is afflicted may feel he is making the greater adjustment. I had to explain to my children, when we received many kindnesses, the difference between Christian brotherhood and charity.

I was also aware of their struggles in accepting my disability as we left church one Sunday morning. Walking with the aid of my crutch, I passed an older acquaintance plodding along behind his walker.

"If you and I were to race," I teased my friend, "I wonder who would win."

My teenagers were horrified. "What poor taste, Mother," they exclaimed later. "Kidding someone about his handicap!" I knew that more than etiquette was involved in the rebuke. My crutch, symbol of what had befallen our family was no joking matter to them.

Those of us who suffer a handicap may face

a concurrent loss of personhood. I struggled with this possibility as I wondered how I, with a crippling disease, could continue to function as a wife and mother.

"But you are still *you*," my husband reassured me.

"In appreciation for what you *are*," a friend signed a letter, and I knew that she, too, was saying that life is a matter of *being* as well as of *doing*.

I have learned to take life in small bites, to live a day at a time, and to appreciate the words of Moses, "As your days, so shall your strength be." Using limited energies wisely calls for simplification of menus and housekeeping procedures; it means eliminating nonessentials and working together with other members of the family.

In my darkest moments, God's love has been strong and warm and His presence a reality. Perhaps the greatest lesson I have learned in the School of Patience is that every day is a gift of God to be treasured and to be lived with joy and abandon.

As for accomplishing my academic goal, I am afraid my diploma in Patience, when I receive it, will have been earned by degrees!

SHE DIGS THE EARTH

WHEN I made my original outline for this book, I had a chapter in mind entitled "My Three Friends and How They Cope." All three ladies have been victims of poliomyelitis since 1952, but their circumstances are vastly different. However, a mutual friend said that she did not like this title, as it did not do justice to the persons involved.

"Those women do more than cope," she pointed out. "They live full and enriched lives."

I had to agree, and the more I talked with

Emma (Mrs. Robert Hartzler), Geri (Mrs. Chester Raber), and Evelyn (Mrs. Royal Bauer), the more sure I became that I must write a chapter on each.

More than twenty years have passed since Emma, Geri, and Evelyn were struck by the polio enemy which had not yet succumbed to the vaccine developed in 1953. Geri and Emma were living in our town of Goshen, Indiana, at the time, but Evelyn was a world away when she became ill. She was on missionary assignment in India.

Emma Hartzler, the busy wife of a pastor, was expecting her third child when she suddenly found herself in a strange new world. A college graduate, Emma often served as secretary to her husband as well as helpmate and friend to the local congregation. And with active sons — Geoff going on six and Greg just eight — dull moments at the Hartzler home were rare.

That particular Saturday in September 1952, Emma remembers waking up with pain in her shoulder and back, not too unusual for a pregnant woman, especially one who had spent the previous day painting baby furniture. That forenoon she took one of the boys to the dentist and found it almost impossible to climb the stairs to his office.

After lunch she stood over a hot dye-kettle stirring baby clothes, then somehow managed to hang them on the line in the backyard before dragging herself back inside. There she collapsed in utter exhaustion on the boys' bottom bunk. Bob checked her temperature — she had no fever, no sore throat, no symptoms except that awful fatigue. But she felt sick, and Bob helped her upstairs to bed.

Then a weird feeling began to creep over Emma's shoulders, slowly down her arms. Bob called the doctor who found her neck slightly stiff. The weird feeling spread down her legs. Shortly after midnight an ambulance sped Emma to the hospital. A spinal tap revealed that Emma had polio, later confirmed as spinal-bulbar polio. By the next day, Emma's breathing became so difficult she had to be rushed into an iron lung.

Five days later, on September 11, Kim arrived — six weeks early. Emma still had enough muscle control to give birth to the baby naturally, but the baby didn't breathe and had to be given emergency treatment. The next day tiny Kim was taken to Bob's sister's home where she and her mother and a pediatrician joined forces to keep the screaming premie alive.

At the Hartzler home Greg and Geoff were being taken care of by friends and by Emma's mother who came from Ohio to help.

Meanwhile, at the hospital, a corps of nurses and doctors and a hall full of praying friends joined Bob in the fight to keep Emma alive. Over the next three weeks her condition steadily worsened, her temperature approached 106 degrees, and she had to undergo a tracheotomy. She became totally paralyzed, even losing her sight for a time.

Her new son was six weeks old before Emma was strong enough for his first visit. For six months she was confined to the iron lung, then was able to take short periods on the rocking bed, which at first made her "seasick."

After 8 1/2 months in the hospital, Emma was moved home with her rocking bed and iron lung. Life had changed radically since the day she was preparing for the coming of the new baby — not only for Emma, but for the entire family. But they were all together again, with Bob's mother moving in to manage the household and help raise the three sons.

Most of Emma's early energies had to be spent in being exercised. Gradually some of her muscles responded and certain abilities returned. Today she is thankful she can read and write, though she cannot handle a needle, sit up, walk, or draw a normal breath.

The March of Dimes was extremely helpful — an absolute lifesaver — during these early months, supplying Emma with the necessary equipment and paying for nursing care and the huge hospital bills. It still furnishes her basic equipment.

I asked Emma what her major problem is. "Fear that the power will go off, as it has on numerous occasions," she replied, "sometimes briefly, sometimes for several hours or more. But help has always been supplied. So far I've survived — though during such traumas I make no claims at coping!"

"I never have trouble finding things to do," she added, "though I sometimes have trouble finding the energy to keep up with my ambitions! I could spend all my time reading, but I also like to be creative, not just entertained. Virtually all I can do really depends on what someone else can do for me. But learning to deal with helplessness comes through learning to accept help. So when it's offered, I accept. And when it isn't, I go the second mile. I ask!

Emma has continued and sharpened her earlier practice of entering contests. Her adeptness at this has won some 300 prizes, including a dishwasher, two washers, a sink, and a water heater, "but mostly little things," she says. She also enjoys writing poetry and has been published in magazines and an anthology, "Indiana Sesquicentennial Poets." At the "Art for Religion Exhibition" in Indianapolis her poetry has won the Laus Tibi Deo award for best of show.

"Right now, though, my 'thing' is the environment," Emma states, adding that she finds it the most challenging of all her projects.

The portholes of her iron lung are decorated with slogans: I Dig Earth; Earth — I Care; Life Is Precious — Death to Pollution; Protect Our Environment.

I and the friends who accompanied me on a visit to Emma smiled as we read these slogans. After complimenting her on her appearance — she coordinates her sheets and blouses — we asked her about a button she was wearing. It read, "Support the Non-Stop Goose."

"I was hoping you'd ask," she smiled. "The poor geese that leave Canada for points south, such as Mexico, are getting short of rest stops." We caught some of her enthusiasm as we listened to her explanation. "Estuaries and wetlands are being endangered by overdevelopment, by tanker spills, by industrial and pesticide pollution, by dredging, by use as dumps. To call attention to the birds' plight, the Young Sierra Club is petitioning the president to develop a jet-propelled goose that won't need to stop! Actually, the goose problem is really our problem. Not only do wetlands shelter migratory birds and other wildlife, but they are essential nurseries in the food production chain of both land and water."

While we listened, we signed several petitions, one of which was a plea to help halt motorcycle damage in Hoosier National Forest. Later we received letters of acknowledgement and appreciation from the congressman to which it was sent.

Emma's interest in preserving the environment and natural resources is more than "busy work" to occupy her time. Although she cannot get closer than her window to view the object of her concern, she really does care. As a member of the Izaak Walton League, Friends of the Earth, Indiana Conservation Council, Indiana Eco-Coalition, The Wilderness Society, National Wildlife Federation, and similar organizations, she has assembled kits of information to distribute to school libraries and friends. She writes to persons of influence and publishes an occasional article.

Over the past weekend she had written short notes of concern on the phosphate issue to twenty-four Indiana Assembly persons. "It is best not to write long, detailed letters because most like to be creative, not just entertained. Virtually all I can do really depends on what someone else can do for me. But learning to deal with helplessness comes through learning to accept help. So when it's offered, I accept. And when it isn't, I go the second mile. I ask!

Emma has continued and sharpened her earlier practice of entering contests. Her adeptness at this has won some 300 prizes, including a dishwasher, two washers, a sink, and a water heater, "but mostly little things," she says. She also enjoys writing poetry and has been published in magazines and an anthology, "Indiana Sesquicentennial Poets." At the "Art for Religion Exhibition" in Indianapolis her poetry has won the Laus Tibi Deo award for best of show.

"Right now, though, my 'thing' is the environment," Emma states, adding that she finds it the most challenging of all her projects.

The portholes of her iron lung are decorated with slogans: I Dig Earth; Earth — I Care; Life Is Precious — Death to Pollution; Protect Our Environment.

I and the friends who accompanied me on a visit to Emma smiled as we read these slogans. After complimenting her on her appearance — she coordinates her sheets and blouses — we asked her about a button she was wearing. It read, "Support the Non-Stop Goose."

"I was hoping you'd ask," she smiled. "The poor geese that leave Canada for points south, such as Mexico, are getting short of rest stops." We caught some of her enthusiasm as we listened to her explanation. "Estuaries and wetlands are being endangered by overdevelopment, by tanker spills, by industrial and pesticide pollution, by dredging, by use as dumps. To call attention to the birds' plight, the Young Sierra Club is petitioning the president to develop a jet-propelled goose that won't need to stop! Actually, the goose problem is really our problem. Not only do wetlands shelter migratory birds and other wildlife, but they are essential nurseries in the food production chain of both land and water."

While we listened, we signed several petitions, one of which was a plea to help halt motorcycle damage in Hoosier National Forest. Later we received letters of acknowledgement and appreciation from the congressman to which it was sent.

Emma's interest in preserving the environment and natural resources is more than "busy work" to occupy her time. Although she cannot get closer than her window to view the object of her concern, she really does care. As a member of the Izaak Walton League, Friends of the Earth, Indiana Conservation Council, Indiana Eco-Coalition, The Wilderness Society, National Wildlife Federation, and similar organizations, she has assembled kits of information to distribute to school libraries and friends. She writes to persons of influence and publishes an occasional article.

Over the past weekend she had written short notes of concern on the phosphate issue to twenty-four Indiana Assembly persons. "It is best not to write long, detailed letters because most best helps in coping over the years has been the assistance of a series of just great teenagers. They give me an hour or two a day, running errands, putting things away, getting things out, opening packages, sewing on buttons, sharpening pencils, cleaning drawers, manicuring my nails, just letting me boss them around and doing a million little things that help me keep my sanity."

During the day Emma answers her own phone (a Swedish Ericaphon, the gift of a Sunday school class) and pursues her projects. She keeps a compact "desk-dressing table-medicine cabinet" box (made for her by Kim) neatly organized and placed beside her on the rocking bed with other materials on a bedside table and in a nearby cupboard. While we visited her, one of us had a problem with a torn nail, and Emma directed her to a drawer labeled "nail clipper."

Then the mailman came into the room, picking up a stack of letters and delivering the incoming correspondence and literature. We were amazed at the volume, not all of which was "junk mail." Emma told us that the mailman arrived one day just as her electric blanket began shooting sparks into the bedside window drapes. He quickly dropped everything, crawled under the rocking bed, and unplugged the smoking blanket!

When Emma's sons were still at home, she joined in the family routine as much as possible. She had a room just off the kitchen, where she often supervised baking projects. The boys and legislators take time only to scan for your opinion," she mentioned, "though sometimes your thoughtful reasoning can be helpful, too. Just write! Study the issues. Know what is going on. Get involved!"

Emma's day begins early, before Bob meets with colleagues over a 6:30 breakfast to start his own workday. After giving her a bath and morning care, he transfers her to her rocking bed, where she stays until suppertime, when he returns from his work as Administrator of Oaklawn Psychiatric Center in nearby Elkhart.

"The lung seems formidable to most people," Emma told us, recalling a little boy at the hospital who spoke of the "lady in the washing machine."

"Do you find it more comfortable than the rocking bed?" we asked.

"Well, yes and no," she replied. "I can breathe easier in the iron lung and can rest and watch TV. But it's not all that comfortable and all I can *do* there is to "think great thoughts" as Bob likes to remind me! I keep a pad and pencil inside to write myself notes to decipher the next day. Just changing back and forth is helpful, however."

She told us that her first TV was made possible by a birthday card and money shower sponsored by some of her friends. Then several years ago a businessman heard of her unsuccessful attempts to win a color set and supplied her with one.

"In addition to the steadfast support of my long-suffering husband and family, one of my their concerns were of great interest to her. "They still are," she affirms.

Emma remembers asking Greg how he felt after first seeing his mother in an iron lung. "He said, 'It was very sad. I felt like crying, but I didn't.' At home he drew a picture of me in the lung to show to me on his next visit."

Today Geoffrey is a resident in Internal Medicine at the Mayo Clinic and Gregory is an attorney in his hometown. ("I wouldn't have a chance in a lawsuit *Hartzler* versus *Brenneman*," I teased.) Both boys have understanding and helpful wives. A pastel portrait of a beautiful brown-eyed baby hangs on the wall in front of Emma's bed — "Our granddaughter, Abigail Melissa," says Emma with grandmotherly pride.

The third son, Kim, the one born after his mother became ill, died suddenly a few years ago of a cerebral hemorrhage. The sense of loss, as for any parent, is not easily described. Kim was sixteen and full of vitality and interest in life.

Thinking of Emma's many difficult experiences — adjusting to remaining confined, regaining her ability to speak, having to depend on others to wait on her for even the simplest necessities of living, and the early death of her youngest child, we asked Emma a hard question.

"What, Emma, has sustained you through all of this?"

She was ready with an answer. "Years ago, when Bob was in seminary in Chicago," she recalled, "we attended a banquet where a speaker made a point which stuck with me. He emphatically exclaimed, 'External pressures be hanged! What about your internal braces?' I remind myself of that advice often and watch out for brace-nibbling termites!"

She has also found consolation in Proverbs 3:6, "In all thy ways acknowledge him, and he shall direct thy paths."

"I used to enjoy playing the piano and singing," Emma went on, "but when one thing is taken from you, you find fulfillment in other things. Not only are there other doors to open, but I find one way to cope is to keep some doors closed. No one can do everything anyway. Limitations simply simplify the choosing."

"In what ways have other people helped?" I asked, wondering about her experiences of brotherhood and sisterhood.

"My sister-in-law was marvelous. She taught school and shared the responsibility for taking care of Kim as well as her own two children. Even so, she visited me every day but one during the entire 8 1/2 months I was in the hospital. And every morning she sent a fresh rose for the tiny vase taped to my iron lung.

"We have always had meaningful support from friends, the church, and the entire community," she went on, and mentioned some outstanding favors. A men's chorus gave the family a home freezer and a parishoner gave them a clothes dryer. "After I had gone from IVs to stomach tube feedings to baby foods to normal diet, I enjoyed surprise treats, too," she continued. "Little gifts and cards give a lift. And flowers — to this day I am seldom without fresh flowers or plants. As long as I couldn't wear my glasses, I liked having Bob read to me, especially from the Book of Psalms. Visitors were always welcome. They still are!

"On Saturdays the boys came to visit me in the hospital," Emma remembered. "They were amazed by the fact that the image in my TV set could be reversed so that it looked right to me in the mirror on the lung. Now my backwards clock intrigues youngsters (and oldsters).

"I've had wonderful nurses who have contributed far beyond the call of duty, nurses of many faiths, but all helping to sustain my faith.

"We're grateful, too, that Bob's mother (now in her late 70's) was willing to take on her second family and has been able to stay with us all these years."

We discussed the fact that Emma's children probably had learned compassion and independence from the difficult side of their lives. Emma related that she tried to join the family for the evening meal and that the boys had taken their turns, along with Bob, in feeding her. They also did their share of dishwashing, floor polishing, errand running, and grocery shopping. As they grew up they had outside jobs, too — from paperboy and lawn mower to stock boy, cashier, musician, factory worker, linotype operator, and the like. They managed to put themselves through college this way.

"Emma," I asked, remembering that even wellintentioned people sometimes do not understand the handicapped, "what did people do along the way which did not help you?"

She hesitated. "Those things have been so rare and so minor — but occasionally a little gossip gets back to me. On one of my visits to the hospital, for instance, word got around that I was pregnant! And, according to gossip, we used polio funds to purchase the freezer! I'm probably too protected to hear anything worse. But I don't think people mean to be hurtful; they're really just interested and concerned."

"Do people forget you?"

"I don't feel forgotten. But people make thoughtless remarks sometimes. One day a lady looked me over and then exclaimed, 'Well, at least you're clean.' A man met Bob on the street and asked, 'Is her mind all right?' A logical question!"

Her mind is definitely "all right," as my friends and I could not help noticing. We were reminded of Eleanor Roosevelt's reply when she was asked if she thought her husband's illness (polio) had affected his mentality. Her answer was, "Yes, anyone who has gone through great suffering is bound to have a greater sympathy and understanding of the problems of mankind."

Someone who has been close to death so many times is bound to appreciate life more fully. (On one occasion Emma reported hearing fantastically beautiful out-of-this-world music — a celestial choir?) We talked about the will to live, the gift of life, how we have varying life-spans, but that all life is precious.

Emma feels that God gave man dominion over all the earth as a sacred trust. We need to exercise tender loving care in its use and not exploit and despoil it. Our "need" and our greed can drive us to destruction, she says.

As we left, we visitors felt like an elderly town character who, before his death, made daily bicycle trips by Emma's window to gaze in at her. We, too, had caught a glimpse of a valiant spirit for whom life, although physically restricted, is nevertheless meaningful, useful, and a joy to others. Although she does not dig the earth with shovel and spade, she "digs" the earth and its resources in the modern meaning of the word dig, determined to make her special contribution to her world and to ours.

MOUNTAINS TO CLIMB

TWO ANXIOUS spouses, Robert Hartzler and Chester Raber, found themselves together in the halls of the Elkhart (Ind.) General Hospital. Already friends, they became closer comrades during the epidemic of poliomyelitis which landed Emma Hartzler and Geri Raber in the polio wards in 1952.

Although Geri was new at fighting the disease in her own body, she had already been involved in the battle against polio. As a young registered nurse she had been assigned to the polio ward just weeks before she became ill herself.

"Did you contract polio while you worked?" I asked Geri one day as we drank coffee together.

"I don't think so," she replied. "In those days it was just in the air, it seemed, and I probably got it like anyone else — in the grocery store or some such place."

While we lunched Geri and I giggled over her recent experience trying to join Chet at a professional meeting in Indianapolis. She had attempted to get on a commuter plane, but found that the only railing was a chain to hang onto. Since Geri walks with the aid of crutches, boarding with only this support would have been impossible. She had to be pushed and pulled on board. After more difficult experiences in the airport, she arrived at her destination, only to find it difficult to convince the motel receptionist that she was really Chet's wife!

"Don't ever take the commuter," she advised me.

I thought of the adventuresome young Geri I had known in school during our youth — how she enjoyed climbing mountains, for instance. Surely she had been climbing mountains symbolically for many years.

We went back to the time when Geri, the young wife of a college student, first found herself in the polio ward.

"I was the last case in Elkhart County," she told me. "The following spring, 1953, a vaccine was finally available."

Then 23 years of age, Geri became ill on the first anniversary of her wedding. She had graduated from a school of nursing and was in the process of helping her husband get his degree. Geri was hospitalized in Elkhart for three weeks, then transferred to a larger institution for another two months. During this time her mother and Chet's mother took turns running her household, which, as yet uncomplicated with children, was not too difficult.

But the mountains to be climbed by Geri were still ahead. Oddly enough, the first obstacle was a physician's advice.

"He wanted to put me in braces or a wheelchair immediately," Geri recalls. "But I learned of another hospital center, in New Hampshire, where the doctor held a different point of view. His approach was, 'Let's see what you *can* do.' Although a certain amount of risk is involved with using crutches, I lead a different kind of life as a result of this doctor's philosophy."

For instance, with her feet strapped to the back pedals of a bicycle-built-for-two, she accompanies her family and friends on long bicycle hikes.

"I think a patient sometimes knows herself better than anyone else and should have some say in these matters," she philosophized. "The patient has to take some initiative. If I had listened only to my first doctor, I would be living with many more limitations."

She recalled that the doctor in New Hampshire gave her good therapy and sound advice. "Do the maximum in your rehabilitation—

but learn when to stop."

A second mountain Geri surmounted came in connection with helping to finance Chet's graduate study in Louisville, Kentucky. Their apartment was up a flight of stairs, but this was not Geri's major problem.

"There I had one of the most traumatic experiences in my life — looking for a job," she recalled. "I learned the struggle a handicapped person goes through in seeking a job. No one was interested in my mind or my skills. I could find nothing in the nursing field until I met the nursing director at a Baptist hospital who said, 'You know, I've been looking for someone like you. But it won't be great pay.'

"I worked, technically, as the hospital's librarian, but actually I was the director's executive secretary. I was able to take a lot of detailed work off her back and at the same time gain some confidence in myself. She'd never had a secretary who understood medical terms, and I knew I was valuable to her. She never knew how valuable she was to me."

Then Chet, who was studying the psychology of religion, returned to a teaching job at Goshen College. That year Geri surmounted another mountain. The good doctor in New Hampshire had encouraged her to have a family. Jon was born in 1955 and 2 1/2 years later Kristin arrived, rounding out their family.

"When we had a second child, people thought we were crazy," Geri mused. "But I figured if I needed help in caring for one, I might as well have help for two." After having an "auntie" for eighteen months when the children were very small, she and Chet managed for years without domestic help.

Now they have a woman for the heavier work. "The help I have needed most is with the weekly housecleaning," she explained. "Chet did most of this for ten years and I thought he deserved a vacation."

Geri can manage cooking for her family, but finds entertaining for meals difficult.

"I do okay with coffee and dessert, where we set things out and people help themselves," she mentioned.

Do her teenagers help? "With some things," Geri said, "but sometimes Kris has so many school and church functions that her help is limited. We try to roll with the punches," she said.

"One thing is very important to me," Geri analyzed. "I had polio before I had children. I had things squared with Chet, and I felt secure with him. I felt secure with my family and friends and adopted a satisfying way of life before the children came. But I feared my children's reaction when they got older. My fears of their embarrassment about me never materialized. I don't feel hardship was imposed on them. Maybe it's because Chet and I don't feel embarrassed. There are things we can't do as a family because I can't do them. But that is just the way it is."

When I interviewed Geri, her daughter Kris was fifteen, Jon eighteen. Chet had worked in a Maryland Mental Health Center for eight years and was now Director of Education at a nearby psychiatric center.

"Chet brings work home at night, as do most professional people, and he has to travel quite a bit," Geri acknowledged. "We accept it."

"Like your other circumstances?"

She laughed, and I was reminded of another observation I had made. "You all seem to have a good sense of humor."

"I think so. Chet and I have fun most of the time, and both children can be clowns."

In spite of Geri's sense of humor, however, she is not without problems, and would be the first to admit it.

"I can't think coping means succeeding all the time," she said thoughtfully. "I think it means managing your life — getting on with what you're planning to do even when you don't feel like doing it. Sometimes this means lowering your goals temporarily and/or permanently."

Geri told me that her housekeeping is not always up to her standards, even with hired help. And, although she would love entertaining in a big way and doing everything "right," she cannot always reciprocate in kind when she is invited out.

"Appearances can be deceiving," she stated. "For some reason I give an appearance of confidence which makes some people think I am always on top. Of course, this is not so. When I had my stomach X-rayed for possible ulcers, a friend remarked, 'Oh no, not you. You're not the type!' People can hardly understand the pressures of a handicapped person when they see him or her only occasionally."

What are Geri's particular problems? "I guess the main problem is that my body can't keep up with my mind. My mind runs ahead of my body's ability to perform. Needing a nap in the afternoon, for instance, is a nuisance to me. Yet, on workdays when I can't fit it in, I'm not good for much in the evening. Then there are transportation problems, especially in the winter months. Although I can drive a car, I cannot safely walk on ice. I don't like making a big deal out of something, as happened that time on the commuter plane."

We talked about persons who say, "You should be thankful things are not worse than they are." This always rankles Geri, since the person speaking is usually in racing form.

We also discussed how other people can be most helpful, and Geri told of a physician's wife who had been a real lifesaver when Geri broke her leg a few weeks before Christmas several years ago. In a matter-of-fact way this friend called Geri and told her she had six hours to give and the use of a car. Geri should be ready for her on Thursday morning with a list of things she wanted to do.

Arriving at the promised time, this busy but caring friend relieved Geri and Chet of many errands and helped Geri feel better prepared for the holidays. It was a kindness she would never forget.

Geri's job, seated by the telephone of a team medical group, is to answer questions for which a doctor is not needed and to channel messages to the proper physcian when more complicated help is required. I asked Geri if she felt that her own circumstances help her to better understand the problems of others.

She answered with conviction, speaking for both herself and Chet, whose job also involves working with people. "I am sure insights we have developed help both of us to do our jobs better," she said, telling of Chet's care for troubled persons, even when they call late at night.

"I know how important it is for people with problems not to feel cut off," she said. "People need many things and surely they need understanding. The hard times in one's own life bring better understanding for other people's troubles."

Geri has learned to accept risk, the support of medical help, and the limitations of her particular handicap. On those days when she works at the doctor's office I can hear confidence and empathy in the tone of her voice as I call her on the telephone.

"This is the nurse," she says. "May I help you . . . ? And suddenly you know that if anyone can help, she can.

THROUGH SUNLIGHT
AND SHADOW

WHEN Evelyn Bauer accompanied her husband, Royal, on evangelistic tours in India, going into villages with the Bible women, she didn't mind camping out in a tent. All her life Evelyn had been an outdoor girl. She grew up in a little town in a Pennsylvania valley called Soap Hollow. Evelyn's mother instilled love of gardens and plants and Evelyn and her friends hiked in all seasons of the year.

Evelyn did not hesitate to take little Stevie along on these evangelistic outings. A breastfed child, Steve fit into the camping program with ease. When he was only four months old, the family spent an entire month on tour.

Evelyn and Royal had been abroad a little more than three years and were on vacation in southern India when Evelyn became ill with polio. At first they thought it was a recurrence of the malaria which hit her every now and then. Headaches, fever, and sore muscles always accompanied malaria. She was taking the usual medication for this malady when she discovered she could not move her toes or walk across the room. Her case progressed quickly. Baby Steve was turned over to missionary friends, while Evelyn was hospitalized 300 miles away. Affected in her arms and her breathing, Evelyn she was placed in an iron lung for three weeks. She believes the lung saved her life.

Although the lung was temporarily crucial to her. Evelyn's goal became breathing for extended periods on her own so she would not be dependent upon the lung.

And it was good that she did learn to breathe independently. Two months after her hospitalization in India, Evelyn was lying on a stretcher across two seats of a commercial plane, headed for home. Accompanied by a physical therapist friend, she returned to her home state to be hospitalized near Pittsburgh for another eight months. At the same time Stevie was placed in the loving hands of his grandmother Showalter.

Evelyn, it was discovered, had not one but two kinds of polio. She gladly cooperated with the not-yet-famous Dr. Jonas Salk, who tried his serum on her. Everyone at the hospital was excited about Dr. Salk's experiments. Although his vaccine was not yet perfected, it seemed he was on the right track.

After her release from the Pittsburgh hospital, Evelyn returned to her parental home, where the family remained for a year during her further recuperation.

For years after Evelyn became ill, she was often asked about her experiences. She found it difficult to share orally, so she began writing down her feelings in what became the book *Through Sunlight and Shadow* (published in 1959 by Herald Press, Scottdale, Pennsylvania). Evelyn wrote the first draft of her book in longhand. After discovering that with her arm in a sling, she could operate an electric typewriter, she typed the second and third drafts. Of the early period of her adjustment to her new circumstances, Evelyn wrote:

> In spite of the advantages in being at home and doing the exercises regularly, the muscles of my legs did not respond. My arms with use continued to make small improvements gradually.
>
> Each change of location brought with it new adjustments which had to be made. It was not easy to watch my mother lovingly working day after day preparing our meals, taking care of our son, and doing many other tasks of which I would have liked to relieve her. I had often been conscience-smitten that I didn't help her more in my earlier years, and now it was too late to help her with her physical work.
>
> It was only natural for Mother to feel sorry for

me because I could not do the many things she knew I had always loved to do. For her to see my difficulties in movement was harder on her than it was on me. She did well in not showing it, but knowing her, I could not help knowing her hurt too. In turn, it was harder for me to endure the thought of her sorrow than it was to bear my own handicaps.

It was too hard to talk about it openly, so I wrote her a note trying to differentiate between pity and love. I wrote that if pity and love could be separated, then "Do not pity me, please — only love me." I tried to point out many of the blessings that God had granted me in order to prove that I truly was not an object worthy of pity.

I considered myself fortunate in many ways. My childhood had been a happy one. My parents had made my college education possible. Our experiences in India were precious, and we hoped had somehow furthered God's cause for man's salvation. Thus the first twenty-five years of my life had been filled so full of happiness and blessings that they would do for a lifetime. Perhaps I have had more happy experiences — more meaningful joys and privileges — than many have in a long lifetime. I wrote Mother that I didn't feel I was missing anything.

When Evelyn discovered that, with her arm in a sling, she could manage a number of activities, a big hurdle was overcome. An art student in college, Evie took another art course by correspondence and enjoyed oil painting and textile painting. Of the latter she wrote:

> I also tried textile painting and found my hand steady enough to cut my own stencils. The first ten dollars I made by painting pillowcases for others was also a great joy to me. During my stay

in the hospital it had been an unpleasant thought that I might be wholly dependent on others. I realized there are handicapped people who have to bear such a position and do it nobly. But I thanked God for the return of a useful right hand.

At one point Evelyn was able to teach a few art courses in a local high school.

Another achievement for Evelyn was the use of her portable electric sewing machine. Having always enjoyed sewing, she learned to push the footfeed with her best hand — her right one — and guide the material with her left. Not only did this make it possible for her to sew most of her own clothes, but to piece bright-colored quilt tops for the sewing group of her church.

Evelyn's present home, a modest, one-story dwelling in Goshen, Indiana, reflects her artistic talents. Flowers and houseplants are skillfully arranged. Evelyn's paintings adorn the walls, and three bookshelves are filled with books which she earned by reviewing them for a denominational press. Several years after the Bauers moved to Goshen, Evie's parents moved there also, taking residence about a block away. When Evelyn's mother died, Evelyn felt the loss of her companionship intensely.

Not long ago Evelyn was asked to speak to a women's group on "God's Grace in Physical Weakness." As she told the group, the request came at a hard time because the efficient household helper they had employed for twelve years was leaving and a replacement was difficult to find.

However, Evie remarked, God's grace is operative in both good and bad times. She documented this by quoting a passage from her book which, although written fifteen years earlier, still summed up her philosophy:

> I can never forget the things that God seemed to whisper to me during the first weeks of my illness. The experience of having the assurance of His love at the very beginning was not just an incident for that one day only. It was so definite and real then, that ever since I am assured that I am in His loving care. I do not believe that God did more for me in showing His love than He does for all His loved ones when they go through times of crisis. That is when He is nearest, if we recognize the fact. As we keep our hearts open to Him, He shows us His love in many quiet ways.
>
> Everyone has troubles of one kind or another in his life on this earth. God lets the rain fall on the just and the unjust. If the rain stands for the natural good things of this life, I think it is true that He allows the natural "bad" things to fall on the just and the unjust also. Troubles, such as loss of loved ones, loss of health, loss of friends, or financial loss, can befall anyone and often nothing can be done to prevent them. For the Christian all such troubles can be blessings because of God's love. I have found it true — He does work all things together for good to those that love Him.

Perhaps Evelyn's philosophy was best expressed in words which she featured in a wall hanging at her and Royal's 25th anniversary celebration. Behind the table at which college son Steve and his fiancee served were the words, "God is good; thank Him."

FROM WHEELCHAIR
TO PIKE'S PEAK

"I MADE IT. I made it. I made it!" There was that look of triumph on Jane Slabaugh's face which her mother had come to recognize after each hard-won success.

This time she'd made Pikes Peak. Other teen friends had also climbed the 14,100-foot peak, and they too were triumphant and somewhat sore. But they hadn't scaled the other peaks that Jane had climbed in recent years.

For only a month had passed since she'd been pronounced cured of dermatomyositis — one of very few persons known to have completely recovered from this disease.

When 9-year-old Jane was diagnosed as having the rare, deteriorating muscle-and-skin disease, she weighed only 54 pounds. Her family had noticed strange symptoms for some time: a tendency to drop things, to fall easily, a difficulty in playing the piano as fast as other pupils her age. Now she ran a temperature every day; her medicine didn't agree with her; her joints had a dark, leathery look. As an outpatient of a large medical center, she was given drugs and ordered to go through a daily regimen of exercises.

"Her chances are slim," one doctor put it kindly. Others came right out with the blunt fact: there is no hope! Doctors suggested that Jane be made as comfortable as possible in bed and wheelchair. If she wanted to go to school and the children would not make fun of her, it would be all right, though time would eventually overtake her and death would come.

Jane had other ideas. Withdraw into a book world? Never! "I couldn't figure out what was wrong with me," she recalls. "I made up my mind I would do everything anyone else could do."

It did not offend Jane to have school friends push her in her wheelchair; she felt honored. But she wasn't content to stay in the chair. She would walk. She'd learn to swim. Slowly, she did.

"If I want my weak side to get better, I'll have to use it," Jane said as she worked at climbing a flight of stairs. "Now how does a 9-year-old figure that out for herself?" a doctor asked. Again and again, doctor friends were surprised at her unusual insights.

"What would you like to do more than anything else — what one thing?" a doctor asked her one day.

"I'd like to turn a somersault," was the quick reply.

"But I can't do that myself," the doctor commented kindly. "And lots of your friends can't do it, either."

It took a great deal of practice and when the thing was accomplished, Jane cried with pain. But it was not long until she was somersaulting her way forward across the 30-foot living room of their farm home and eventually making the trip backward the other direction. After that there was a round trip each morning in order "not to be stiff at school."

Doctors said that because of skin complications Jane should stay out of the sun. But her mother would find Jane time after time sunbathing, having stolen out the window to the family's back porch roof.

When Jane first started back to school, her high school brother helped her on and off the school bus. Then this brother won a trip to Chicago and had to be gone for several days. Jane was thrilled to discover that she could get on and off the bus by herself. After that she refused help.

With each accomplishment Jane's mother recalls a special look which came across her face

— a special smile. As she worked at the grueling and often monotonous exercises, Jane would say, "Let's do it one more time." The one more time often brought a small triumph, a link in the chain of successes which eventually climaxed in her recovery. Miraculously, the day arrived when the doctors, who had years before given up hope, pronounced Jane cured. She was 14.

Jane's will to live — to be a part of life — had much to do with her recovery, but as one doctor told her, "You had help from a Higher Power." Jane had many praying friends not only among people she knew personally, but among strangers who'd meet her on the street and assure her of their prayers.

"Everybody — friends, ministers, and especially my parents — had a lot to do with helping me get well," she says. "They all had a lot of patience and love for me that made me want to work and live."

I first learned to know Jane at a contest put on by the Singer Company in which my daughter was also a contestant. Jane, 17, won the local 1966 prize for her age group as she modeled a two-piece suit with matching beret and other accessories which she designed and constructed. With the same outfit she'd won 4-H acclaim.

Her suit took her to Singer's state contest where she won a sewing machine and qualified for national competition. Jane had just returned from a trip to Mexico with fellow students from her high school.

She later was a junior leader in 4-H; secretary of her senior class at Millersburg High

School near Goshen, Indiana; co-editor of her school annual; and a member of a good will club.

"Always on the go — a typical teenager," her mother smiled. "Even a little sassy at times."

After the sewing contest one of Jane's teachers suggested that she might be able to earn a great deal of money with her sewing ability.

"But I don't want to earn a lot of money," Jane responded. "I want to serve people." And that is what Jane has done since she made that statement. Now Mrs. Jerry Derstine, Jane graduated from college, prepared for teaching home economics, and with her husband served in Voluntary Service assignments in a teen center in Mississippi and in Aspen, Colorado, where she worked as a volunteer teacher's aide.

"God had a reason to let me live," Jane said. "Now I should live for Him and do what He wants me to do. He gave me a life, and I want to give it back to Him."

WHEN GOD DOES NOT HEAL

Guest Chapter by Katie Funk Wiebe

THE HUSBAND of a friend of mine had been ill for some time. In keeping with the Scripture in James 5, the family called the minister and deacons of the church, who anointed the sick man with oil and prayed for his healing. A week later he died.

I listened quietly to the comments of friends and acquaintances discussing the man's death. Some wondered kindly yet skeptically what kind of Pollyanna faith would deny the realities of life and expect God to heal a disease for which the doctors had no cure. Others wondered lovingly yet somewhat bewildered: when people pray in faith and God does not heal, is that faith vain? Is the death of a loved one the reward for putting one's faith in Him? How does one still the questioning of one's own soul after such an experience?

Today's renewed interest in and study of spiritual healing is offering hundreds of sick people hope of recovery as this movement gains impetus. Yet it is also leaving in its wake perplexed persons who wonder what the magic formula for healing may be. And, if there is one, why can't they learn to say the right words?

I have long agreed with the late V. Raymond Edman that certain spiritual experiences should remain a secret between the believer and his Lord and need not be blurted out in testimony upon demand. For years I have kept to myself the deep feelings regarding my late husband's illness and death. Yet as I sense the questions of people thrust into similar experiences I feel free to speak. Perhaps a little of what I write may help a person who wonders why he or one of his has not been healed.

The fall of 1958 is permanently etched in my memory. Our family had just arrived in Ontario from Saskatchewan after experiencing a dry, rather unpleasant summer there. Scorched grass had struggled in front yards to remain alive and loose dust swirled about one's every step. Compared to the meager garden returns in Saskatchewan the bountiful produce of the

Niagara Peninsula seemed the firstfruits of Eden. Everywhere we saw green grass. Trees towered into the heavens instead of crouching like tired old people. Flowers bloomed brilliantly. If this was Ontario, we were going to love it.

We had come from a small pastorate in the prairies to teach in a private high school and at the same time continue my husband's education. I felt almost like my immigrant mother some 35 years earlier, who with husband and two small children had thankfully left everything behind in Russia to make a new home and life in Canada.

The first week of school was disappointing and difficult. The first weekend Walter, my husband, lay ill, doubled up with a pain in his abdomen. His illness was generally diagnosed by the doctor as flu. The pain in his abdomen subsided, but the general malaise continued week after week. Each new day in the Promised Land became an agony with no apparent medical help.

Four months later when Walter was 1,500 miles away for a church board meeting, his condition suddenly worsened and an emergency operation revealed a ruptured appendix, badly infected. Many people prayed for his recovery. After hanging between life and death for several days, he showed hope of recovery, but the convalescence was slow because of the long time the infection had preyed on his system.

Little did we know that we had begun the first of a series of operations in a fight for his physical life and the first in an even stiffer, battle for spiritual survival. The year had been a fiasco, but as health returned, we made plans to pick up the tangled threads of our life.

A little over a year later when Walter took a routine physical examination for graduate school entrance, the doctors discovered a growth in his abdomen. Because he seemed in generally good health, the operation was postponed until the close of the school year. We clung to the promise, "As thou goest the way shall be opened up before thee step by step."

The diagnosis after the operation was "non-malignant but with danger of recurrence." We were thankful. We praised God for this word from the doctors. To us it was a signal to live again. And we did. We went camping to Algonquin Park to enjoy the haunting shriek of the loons and the grumpy croak of the bullfrogs. Later that summer a third operation was performed, but again we trusted God's Word that when we passed through the waters He would be with us (Is. 43:1-5), and He was.

Walter returned to the university to prepare for his work as a religious journalist, an interest and ambition which had been his since I first met him. Yet as the winter wore into spring, we knew that the disease was once again recurring. By July, he was again confined to the hospital. As I look back upon these days and the weeks following I remember best the times we spent searching the Word of God. We were in need — great physical need and deeper spiritual need. As we read the Gospels together we noticed how Christ was always concerned with the whole man as He ministered to the people.

As we read there was born in us a hope, a trust in God that what He had done in the past, He was also able to do today. Friends encouraged us, sometimes with bold assurance, to pray for healing. It seemed so certain. Surely God's will was health, since He is the Great Physician.

And yet we were human and doubted as we believed. We knew a new growth was constricting the large intestine, but in view of Walter's past medical history the doctors were reluctant to operate. Without surgery the future remained uncertain and each new small symptom of ill health caused dark clouds of fear to descend.

The next weeks were some of the longest we had faced yet as we debated with ourselves, with the doctors, and with God which way we should go. How quickly would the illness progress? Since his condition was rare and the prognosis indefinite, we proceeded with earlier plans to move to Hillsboro, Kansas. To wait for death was to die by slow torture. To do nothing was to rot. I heard later of a patient with a similar disease who lived eleven years.

Walter took a position as book editor in our denominational publishing house. Again and again we prayed for trust. We wanted God to be the groundstuff of our lives, even though we felt at times like the Israelite who "walked in darkness and had no light." Let such a person "trust in the name of the Lord, and stay upon his God," wrote the prophet Isaiah to comfort the exiled Jews. Walter wrote in his journal, "When this illness began I said, "Lord,

You are pushing us into a corner — but as long as Thou art in the corner with us...'"

The corner was to get even tighter. After about seven weeks in his new job, health became an issue once again. Not as a desperate measure to manipulate God, but in obedience to God's Word, we called the elders of the church, who anointed him with oil and prayed over him.

Soon after that he called me from the office one day to say he felt sick. I took him to the hospital. The memory I cherish most even today is the sight of Walter as he drew our three-year-old son to him and murmured, "My little boy." At our last family devotion, as he lay on the living room couch, we sang, "As we walk with the Lord in the light of His Word, what a glory He sheds on our way." Was this the way of glory? He died a few days later.

The faith that God was with us had supported us through a long, difficult period. We had been subject to fears, to anguish, to desperation. Yet when I walked out of the hospital that early Saturday morning to tell the children the long struggle was over, the trust God had given me through weeks and months of difficult living remained with me — not as a strong blinding light, but as a glimmer of hope in the gathering darkness.

At times thereafter I was plagued with the unanswered questions of why God had not healed. Those who had encouraged us to pray for healing now remained silent. Had we been the deluded victims of fanaticism? Had our faith been vain? I don't think so.

I will always be grateful to the kindly old minister, wise in the ways of God and man, who is now himself an invalid, who said to me one day, "The greater miracle than healing today is the faith in those left behind to continue life." Man's greatest need in sickness or in health is a living bond with God. If healing takes place, how tempted some people might be to trust, not in God, but in the experience of healing. Every experience with God of nonhealing becomes a part of one's life, as well as the experience of healing.

Those connected with the sick person can react to nonhealing with faith or with bitterness. God is not defeated because someone dies; we need not be either, nor do we need to resort to the verbal juggling which prompts some people to say after a person dies that "God raised him from his sickbed — He raised him higher."

I believe God can and does heal the sick today. He is on the side of life and health. Yet faith that believes that God is able to heal is not sufficient. As one person said, most Christians, especially those who are seriously ill, do not find it difficult to believe that God who originally gave life to man also has the power to prolong it by healing. To believe that God is able is perhaps the smallest obstacle to healing.

I believe also that healing faith is not the kind that is brought into existence by our zeal, earnestness, or even our presumption. No preacher can promise healing nor can we force ourselves by sheer willpower or intellectual strength to accept this stance. Healing is not something that can be appropriated in desperation. Asserting the words of faith boldly does not bring healing.

The prayer of faith that heals is a gift of God (1 Cor. 12:9), a gift we cannot call into being, and most certainly a gift which is not evoked by learning magic codes. Was this gift the faith the Apostle James wrote about? In his epistle he did not indicate that the Lord would always heal. If so, churches would have the biggest business going. Death would be obliterated and our old folks' homes overpopulated. Yet no one should be discouraged from praying for healing or from going to the skills of medical science. Both are gifts of God.

Healing faith demands total commitment to God and His will whether for health or not. Such faith gives a person strength to face the vicissitudes of life and move on even though the question may often come, "Lord, if you had been here, my brother had not died." Faith does not keep us from ugliness of life — its sin, sorrow, misery, ill health. It gives us power to move on.

When the picture of life is completed, and we see the whole, if we have trusted in Him, not in faith, we find that there was a purpose for every experience and it was good. At the present moment we see a difficult experience as the end of everything. The disciples saw the cross as the end of Jesus' life and ministry when it was the beginning of a new kingdom.

Many years earlier at the death of a favorite teacher, Dr. A. H. Unruh, Walter wrote about life under the sun as being but a fragment: "It never attains perfection, fulfillment, full attainment. Is there a completeness about infancy, childhood, youth, man, the aged? Does life flower, come to a perfect cycle, or does it break off? Why should Dr. Unruh with his wisdom and experience now break off? He is only ready to begin."

The absurdities, the complexities about life can only be answered with continued faith that God will put the fragments together. "A measure of faith is whether you can look at life's darkness and yet believe in the light."

PROFESSIONAL ADVICE FROM A PARALYZED PSYCHIATRIST

ALL MY life I have enjoyed interviewing interesting people, asking them all kinds of questions about their experiences. As I thought over the outline for this book, I had a desire to interview a psychiatrist about the needs of handicapped persons. Since I was acquainted with Dr. Otto Klassen, of nearby Oaklawn Psychiatric Center, I asked his opinion of a professional counselor whom I could speak to on this subject. His answer: "The most qualified person I can think of lives in California. He is Dr. Geroge

Dillinger, and he knows the problems from both the professional and the handicapped perspectives."

Dr. Klassen explained that Dr. Dillinger, with whom he had interned, had met with a serious accident which paralyzed him up to his shoulders. He had nevertheless finished his internship and gone into practice.

I prefer eyeball-to-eyeball interviews, since almost as much can be learned by observing the person interviewed as by his answers to one's questions. And interaction is always preferable in conversation.

But since neither Dr. Dillinger or I could travel easily, and funds were limited, and half a nation lay between us, I decided to try a tape recorder interview. I wrote Dr. Dillinger with my request.

"I tend to have a totally different view in regard to disability," he warned me in his response. "I see everybody as having some sort of disability. So I tend to view the problem from a broad perspective as opposed to zeroing in on an obvious physical deformity."

Nevertheless, Dr. Dillinger stood ready to help in any way he could. To show him that I agreed with him, I sent him a quotation from my earlier book, *The House by the Side of the Road:* "One thing which has helped me to accept my particular handicap is the knowledge that everyone has his own limitations. . . . People with perfectly good legs often hurt on the inside." I also explained that since I have written for particular groups of people, such as expectant and new mothers, I would like to particularize his advice for the physically handicapped.

That settled, Dr. Dillinger and I had the following conversation, courtesy electronic devices and Uncle Sam:

Question: Dr. Dillinger, tell us about the disaster which resulted in your becoming paralyzed and how you have learned to cope with life in spite of your limitations.

Answer: I was thrown out of an automobile in December of 1953, suffering a fracture dislocation of the sixth and seventh cervical vertebrae. At the time I was halfway through my internship. It took me approximately six months to get out of the hospital, and about two months later I returned to finish my internship on a part-time basis. I have used a wheelchair since that time, and simply kept at it, doing everything I could and using my ingenuity as much as necessary. Hospital personnel were most cooperative. I have almost full use of my hands so that I have been able to function quite well in my practice. It is mainly a problem of providing myself with suitable space, with room to move around.

I have worked very hard at trying to be as realistic as possible. In some ways, I have developed a super-sense of what is real and what isn't. I have never stopped looking for ways to increase my abilities, but at the same time I try to recognize realistically what my limitations are. I am always careful to define my exact limitations at the moment. I do not feel this has to be a static condition. My condition may change for the better or worse at any time.

Question: Dr. Dillinger, I see a major problem for persons such as you and for myself. We learned self-help when we were still preschoolers. Suddenly we must shift from degrees of independence to degrees of dependence.

An example of this is loss of the use of the small muscles of the fingers so that we need help with buttoning, tying shoes, and the like. Bigger adjustments are having to give up driving a car or managing other living skills independently. How can we make these adjustments gracefully? How can we fight the feeling that we are a "burden" to others?

Answer: The problem I see in shifting levels of dependency has to do with the emotional attitudes that are attached to these various states. Different people have tremendously different ideas as to what dependence and independence mean to them. The ability to make the adjustments gracefully, as you put it, comes from the acceptance and understanding of the many different normalities of feeling that can be associated with the dependency-independency conflict.

Question: Is it possible that we might become too dependent on other persons so that we might indeed limit their lives and keep them from becoming all that they would like to be?

Answer: I think one is too dependent either when one is not doing all he can and therefore expecting too much of someone else, or when one's demands are excessive in terms of the other person's own limitations. One should be as perceptive of this as possible, but I feel the other people have an equal responsibility to say when they are feeling overly burdened.

Question: How can we know when family members are feeling this tension?

Answer: The main problem that I have observed is when family members get overly involved with a handicapped person, feeling that they have to do more than is possible or is necessary. They have to be reminded that they still have to look after themselves.

Another way of coming at this problem is to challenge the idea which a person has of his particular role in the family, to find out exactly what the family member sees as his role and what are the other possibilities.

Question: In relating to other members of the family, I often wonder how easy I am to live with. I sometimes say that I am a *household administrator*, which lends dignity to my calling. This, being interpreted, means *boss*, but being further interpreted by members of the family, sometimes means *nag*. It is difficult to wait for others to do tasks which, under other circumstances, one would do immediately. How do we cope with negative feelings, especially when we don't feel on top physically?

Answer: I have been irritated at others many times. For me, it is a matter of allowing myself permission to get irritated once in a while. For a number of years I was extremely depressed and often felt like giving up. I received a lot of help by getting into psychiatric therapy, and gradually, over the years, I learned to accept myself more and to feel less resentful about my limitations.

Question: What do you see as the meaning of *acceptance?* I think I have accepted my state. Yet, when my condition changes, I find that I must adjust all over again.

Answer: For me, acceptance is the act of saying that whatever I am at a given moment, no matter what I am feeling, is okay. This, I feel, is an extraordinarily creative act. People shouldn't worry that this act has to be repeated as circumstances change. The reason I say that is because each time the act of acceptance is performed the ability to do so can be strengthened.

Question: Are there unhelpful or wrong ways of coping? Recently when working with a physical therapist, I found myself cheating by using muscle No. 749 when I should have been using No. 153. I believe the therapist calls this "substituting," and when I do this I am doing more harm than good in my exercises. Is it possible that we cheat psychologically, while trying to cope with our problems?

Answer: As far as cheating is concerned, I think this is a highly individual question, and one that can be answered only by the individual himself. I know that it happens a lot; I have done it myself. And I see a lot of other people doing it. In the final analysis we are only cheating ourselves. However, I know many people who cannot face their problems that easily, and that's okay too. But, failing to face themselves honestly, they will be much more limited.

Question: I am concerned about the need for handicapped persons to feel productive. Not long ago, when I was in the hospital for tests, I received many flowers. However, after I came home I received another bouquet from an intuitive friend. The card read, "You received other flowers because you are sick. I send these because you are productive. Congratulations on publishing your new book!"

How fortunate we are if we have something to do to make us feel worthwhile. Do you have any advice along this line?

Answer: I don't think I am particularly fortunate in having a profession. I think I would have felt productive anyway. Finding something which is productive to do is built into all people and is there to be developed. People cop out on this level very easily, and if they're physically handicapped, they come up with even better excuses. I feel that if someone is not being productive, something has gone wrong with him or her. We'd better find out why they're shutting themselves off.

Dr. Dillinger put in one answer to a question I hadn't asked, and I was most happy that he did. He said, "I noticed that you used the word *disaster*. When I was injured my family felt that the accident was a terrible disaster. Some of them still do. However, as the years progressed I have learned so much about myself and other people through my injuries that I can hardly call the event a disaster. When I first began having thoughts like this, I thought that perhaps I was rationalizing all these terrible things that have happened to me. But as I have delved into this line of thinking, I can assure you that I am not rationalizing.

"I certainly wish that there had been easier ways to learn all that I know now. People do not need to feel sorry for themselves when something like this happens if they find the courage to *use* it as a means for looking further into themselves. If they do this, they will find a kind of reward which cannot be gotten in any other way."

I agree with Dr. Dillinger's comments and am grateful he allowed me to share them with you in this chapter.

THE USES OF ADVERSITY

IN A MUSEUM in California our family examined an old stagecoach. Even more interesting than the coach itself were the rules for traveling in this vehicle, clipped from the *Omaha Herald* of 1877 and posted on the wall behind it:

> The best seat inside a stage is the one next to the driver. Even if you have a tendency to seasickness when riding backwards, you'll get over it and will get less jolts and jostling. . . .

In cold weather, don't ride with tight-fitting boots, shoes, or gloves. When the driver asks you to get off and walk, do so without grumbling. He won't request it unless absolutely necessary. If the team runs away, sit still and take your chances. If you jump, nine out of ten times you will get hurt.

In very cold weather abstain entirely from liquor when on the road, because you will freeze twice as quickly when under its influence. Don't growl at the food received at the station, stage companies generally provide the best they can get. Don't keep the stage waiting. Don't smoke a strong pipe in the coach. Spit on the leeward side. . . .

Don't swear or lop over neighbors when sleeping. Take small change to pay expenses. Never shoot on the road as the noise might frighten the horses. Don't discuss politics or religion. Don't point out where murders have been committed, especially if there are women passengers. Don't lag at the washbasin. Don't grease your hair, because travel is dusty.

Don't imagine for a moment that you are going on a picnic. Expect annoyances, discomfort, and some hardship.

Today, when we think of taking a trip, we are likely to envision packing the family luggage in the trunk of a new Buick or enplaning on a jet for a distant city. I love flying. I always feel on top of all my problems and handicaps. Everyone — the booking agent, aircap, and the stewardess — go out of their way to be helpful, and I love food served on planes! But I'm afraid the stagecoach passenger had more of an idea of the hardships on life's journey. He knew that life was no picnic!

Jesus deceived no one who wanted to be His follower. He said, "Birds of the air have nests;

but the Son of man has nowhere to lay his head. . . . In the world you have tribulation; but be of good cheer, I have overcome the world." The Apostle Paul continued in Jesus' realistic tradition when he said, "Expect your share of suffering. . . . Endure hardness, as a good soldier of Jesus Christ."

In other words, we may just as well accept hard times. They are going to come. But there are resources available if we are open to them.

E. Stanley Jones, in his spiritual autobiography, *Song of Ascents,* points out that we are to *use* difficulties, not simply to endure them. One of his illustrations is the quarrel, which can be a means of better understanding between two people if it is properly used. I recently heard a speaker point out that conflict is of the essence of any marriage, since both parties are human, but what results from conflict is dependent upon how it is managed.

I sometimes find it difficult to see any good use for certain musical atrocities (in my opinion) which are committed on our family record player and which, if I don't close my study door, have a tendency to broaden the generation gap. But while I was contemplating this theme, a voice from one of these records quoted the familiar words of Shakespeare found in *As You Like It,* "Sweet are the uses of adversity." So some good use can come even from the airing of the younger set's prized recordings!

At the time when life presents its more serious and unexpected obstacles, it is hard to see how God wants us to use a particular perplexing circumstance. The uses of adversity do not seem sweet when adversity comes. A friend for whom music is an integral part of her very person, as well as her lifework and best form of service, discovered one terrible day that she had a tumor on a vocal chord. Facing the possibility of an altered singing voice, Romaine discovered that it was difficult to integrate her emotions with her faith and intellect.

One day she remembered how her grandfather had developed cataracts at such an advanced age that surgery seemed unwise. Knowing the risks of surgery, he commented, "I want to see what God can teach me through blindness."

Turning the matter over to God, Romaine realized that it might be necessary for her to learn what God could teach her through silence. And even before the surgery she was learning some new dimensions of faith and the tremendous support experienced through the prayers of her friends. "I became aware that my friends were reinforcing and supporting me in a way I had never experienced," she said.

When a difficult experience comes to us — a crisis in our health, loss of job or insecurity about our future, problems in broken relationships or in guiding our children in paths which will lead to joy and not destruction, or personal failures, which are the hardest to take — our first response is to cry out, "Oh no, not me! Oh God, why?" This cry of despair is not sin if only we do not stay on that plateau indefinitely. As we turn our eyes toward God, we are given the insight to ask how we can use this unsolicited circumstance to grow and to glorify Him.

But suffering is still suffering, and we need not whitewash it. Negative thoughts can be beautiful, a counselor says, if they pave the way for positive ones. Another counselor says, "We would not scold our child for running a fever. We would look for the cause. Likewise, we must not scold a loved one for anger. Anger is the emotional temperature and merely shows that there is something deeper which needs attention."

History is filled with illustrations of persons who have overcome adversity or who have even used it for great achievements. Martin Luther King wrote, "My personal trials have taught me the value of unmerited suffering. As my sufferings mounted, I soon realized that there were two ways that I could respond to my situations; either to react with bitterness or seek to transform the suffering into a creative force."

A theologian friend, Millard Lind, says, "Suffering is not meaningless. It is the incarnation of God into our circumstances."

The Bible and other literature tell of many persons who have lived fruitful lives in spite of circumstances which they would never have chosen for themselves. Making sweet uses of adversity, they have surmounted obstacles, borne hardships, endured injustices, overlooked hostilities, forgiven mistreatment and misunderstanding, lived and worked in spite of it all.

For some reason four-letter words have gained for themselves a dubious reputation, but some of the most helpful words in the English language are composed of four letters. Here are six good four-letter words which may help us to conquer those problems with which we have to cope.

(1) *Pray*. The importance of this word cannot be overemphasized, for without it the other five may fall flat. I would not want to cross the street or go to bed at night without having a word with my caring Father.

(2) *Give*. Those of us with a handicap may not be able to serve in some ways for which we would have natural inclination, but we often have more time for listening to and bearing the burdens of others whose handicaps may be more disabling than a physical malady. We give of ourselves when we take time to listen.

(3) *Love*. Our youth remind us often of our unloves, of our tolerances which make pretense of being love, of our inconsistencies in practicing what we so readily preach on the subject. But when we do not love, we cheat ourselves of a creative force which could make a great deal of difference in facing our own situations. When we truly love another, we see in him our own predicament and empathize more than sympathize. For when we are busy loving and caring, we have less time for self-pity, the enemy of all ability to cope.

If we feel misunderstood by those we love most, it helps to remember that they have not experienced our special problems and that they are often carrying heavy burdens of their own. I like to think of Jesus' prayer, when He was so desperately misunderstood, "Father, forgive them, for they know not what they do."

Pehaps we could rephrase this for our own needs: "Father, forgive him for he cannot really understand how I feel"; "Father, forgive him, for he is under pressure or is himself hurting"; "Father, forgive her, for she is tired."

(4) *Work*. Our work may not be of our choosing, but we must have goals and purposes which fit into our limitations and abilities. There are some chores which I reserve for my weakest moments — physically, that is. A telephone call to a discouraged friend, writing out a schedule for family activites, thinking through needs and concerns for those we love, reading (in my case, listening to Talking Books for the Blind) — these are chores which give purpose to life when I cannot scrub floors.

(5) *Cope*. This is the word which inspired this book, a beautiful little word with great potential. One day a friend asked me over a cup of coffee, "How do you stand it, to be so handicapped for such a long time?"

"Well," I answered thoughtfully, "what are the options, the alternatives? Let's see, I could jump off a bridge, but then who would take me there?"

She laughed. "And when you got to the bridge, you wouldn't be able to jump."

"Right. So I guess I'll just have to cope."

(6) *Hope*. But there are those days when we do not cope, or at least not very well. For me, this often happens when I drop off the plateau to which I and my family have become accus-

tomed. Or when circumstances develop within my family or other relationships to complicate my physical problems. At times like this, when we cannot *cope*, we must *hope*.

An acquaintance who was going through a severe trial which chipped away at his self-image and very personhood, awoke one morning with the firm knowledge that God really did love him dearly. It is impossible for us to move outside the encompassing warmth of the love of God, even though there are days when we are not aware of it. Faith, after all, is the knowledge of things *not seen* but nevertheless real and present.

A theologian friend, C. Norman Kraus, spoke one Sunday morning from Luke 24:49 about Christ's challenge to His disciples just before He left the earth: "And behold, I send the promise of my Father upon you; but stay in the city, until you are clothed with power from on high."

He told us that the word "stay" literally means to "sit" and, bringing the expression up to date, we might say, "Sit tight while you wait for the power of God." Perhaps it was because most of my waiting in hope must be done in a sitting position that this rendition of the verse stuck with me. All week I thought of the admoninition to *sit tight*. A feeling of expectancy pervaded my thinking that week.

But on another occasion, when I told a friend on the phone about my uneasiness in connection with a week full of meaningful work ahead she ended our conversation with the words, "hang loose." I pondered how I could combine the two concepts of sitting tight while waiting in hope, and hanging loose so that things would not get me down. I concluded that the ideas were not mutually exclusive. While we are waiting in expectancy, we remind ourselves that our hope is in God, and that nothing which comes our way is of our own doing. We are not *uptight* while we *sit tight*. We can relax while we wait for the promises of God to be fulfilled.

When it is hard to cope let's seize some of God's promises which we can experience in hope: *"All things work together for good to them that love God. . . . Be of good cheer; I have overcome the world. . . . Casting all your care upon him, for he careth for you. . . . Nothing can separate you from the love of God which is in Christ Jesus, your Lord. . . . When he hath tried me, I shall come forth as gold."*

> Yet through all,
> We know this tangled skein
> is in the hands of One
> who sees the end
> from the beginning;
> He shall unravel all.
> — *Alexander Smith*

THE AUTHOR

Born in Harrisonburg, Virginia. Helen Good Brenneman spent her childhood near Hyattsville, Maryland, a suburb of Washington, D.C. She studied at Eastern Mennonite and Goshen colleges, and worked for four years as a clerk in the U.S. Department of Agriculture. Always interested in writing, Helen longed as a girl to become a newspaper reporter, but later found herself writing numerous articles, stories, women's inspirational talks, and devotional books.

Following her marriage to Virgil, the couple served a year in a refugee camp operated by the Mennonite Central Committee in Gronau, Germany, before going to Goshen, Indiana, where her husband studied for the ministry. They served for ten years in two pastorates, at Iowa City, Iowa, and Goshen, Indiana.

Virgil is presently executive secretary of Mennonite Camping Association and a regional representative of International Students, Inc.

Helen and Virgil are the parents of Don, married to Beth Sequin; Lois (known as Tobi), married to Joe Goldfus; John, living at home; and Becky, temporarily employed in Tucson, Arizona.

Helen is author of *Meditations for the New Mother, But Not Forsaken, My Comforters, Meditations for the Expectant Mother, The House by the Side of the Road, Ring a Dozen Doorbells,* and *Marriage: Agony and Ecstasy.* Two of her books have been translated into Spanish, one into German, and another into Portuguese.